GUIDED IMAGERY/ HYPNOTHERAPY

For Healthcare:

We Can Make a Difference

By Linda Bennett, MS, CCHt, LC and
Gisele Marasca-Vargas, CCHt, CLC, CWP

Cover Design and Book Layout by
Gisele Marasca-Vargas

DEDICATION

To all the individuals working to make a difference in today's healthcare…

TABLE OF CONTENTS

FOREWORD by Dan Dziadura

I love physical therapy. There's a certain satisfaction in knowing I help patients minimize pain, maximize strength, and, ultimately, live life with more confidence. Like a detective looking for clues, I was trained to systematically observe and evaluate various parts of the body to determine sources of weakness and limitation, and to prescribe a specific set of exercises and activities to address the concerns. I would be the guide who helped people take ownership of their health and well-being.

At least in theory.

One morning, over 25 years ago, as I was working in a busy hospital in Brooklyn, New York, I was treating two patients who had recently undergone total knee replacement surgery. I couldn't help but notice the striking difference in outcomes that was unfolding. Despite the pain, one patient bit her lip (metaphorically) and stoically bore weight on her surgical leg almost immediately after surgery. In no time, she was walking with an assistive device, tolerating exercise and passive stretching to her knee, and was soon discharged home to resume her life with a new, pain-free, and arthritis-free knee. A successful outcome! The other patient, in obvious distress after her surgery, moaned in agony, resisted standing even with the support of parallel bars, and refused all attempts to walk. I explained to her the importance of physical therapy and of fighting through the pain. Consciously, she understood and agreed, but despite being medicated for pain, she was unable to overcome her fear. She was eventually discharged to a skilled nursing facility to continue her rehab, delaying her discharge home–and a successful outcome–by weeks.

What happened? I put my clinical detective skills to work to diagnose the situation: here were two patients who had the same surgery, on the same day, performed by the same surgeon, using the same type of equipment, and other than some minor differences in medical history (elective orthopedic surgeries are generally done on patients who are otherwise healthy) resulted in two vastly different outcomes.

Obviously, the answer wasn't strictly physical. A major portion of the process was psychological–even subconscious–given that the second patient understood and agreed that she needed to work through her pain and fear but was unable to do so. I knew instinctively that I needed to find a straightforward and evidence-based way to overcome the kind of resistance shown by the second patient, but the answer seemed outside of my professional scope, and therefore, escaped my grasp.

Many years later, as a Rehab department director at a hospital in Phoenix, I was leafing through a catalog to find a coaching program that would help me better support my team of therapists. Instead, my eye was drawn to another item that seemed much more intriguing. The catalog was from SWIHA - Southwest Institute of Healing Arts, and the program was Hypnotherapy. I felt goosebumps when I considered that, as a physical therapist accustomed to treating people's bodies, I could learn the secrets of the mind and potentially find the key to unlock the mysterious resistance demonstrated by that suffering patient many years ago, and by extension, all suffering patients. At SWIHA, I found in Linda Bennett a kind and kindred soul who, as I saw it, gave people tools to help them stop their own suffering. After completing my Medical Hypnotherapy certificate, Linda and I got to work creating the program you'll read about in this book. Along the way we were almost tripped up by dozens of details, but, as Gisele Marasca-Vargas expertly explains, these details are minor bumps that, when crossed, lead down a road of passion, compassion, relief, and freedom.

I'm proud to be part of the important work of re-integrating mind and body to create a new paradigm for Western healthcare. In the capable hands of people like Linda and Gisele, we have a bright future of healing ahead of us.

Dan Dziadura PT, DHSc, MSPT
Director of Rehabilitation Services, and Wellness Coordinator
Phoenix, Arizona

FOREWORD by Robert F. Otto

In today's society, Guided Imagery/Hypnotherapy as a modality of care is well recognized by the general public and the Health Professions.

If we are to gain acceptance in the health/wellness field, results matter. Consistently good results happen when you have a broad knowledge base and apply that knowledge in an organized, standardized manner, while considering the client/patient's goal as priority on the scale of importance. When you follow this recommendation, you'll most often find the results "noteworthy."

This is precisely what occurred in the Guided Imagery/Hypnotherapy volunteer initiative that Linda Bennett and Dan Dziadura implemented at a major regional hospital in Arizona. This book shares the results of the pilot study and tips on how hospitals and clinics around the country can start their initiative.

Guided Imagery/Hypnotherapy continues to show promise. Mounting evidence supports its efficacy as a safe and effective adjunct to conventional medicine for several conditions. Medical professionals today are cautiously optimistic and rising to take notice of the profound effects of Guided Imagery/Hypnotherapy as a cost-effective, non-invasive healing modality in the medical community. This is largely due in part to those who have taken the initiative to memorialize their findings for the sake of future generations. Gathering data through research is paramount to aligning our services with the healthcare field, improving our image, and gaining acceptance in the medical community.

I am delighted to see the continuation of studies in our field and encourage readers to consider doing their part in helping the profession by starting their own initiative in their demographic locale. Future generations are depending on it.

Robert F. Otto, Speaker, Author, President and CEO of the IMDHA - International Medical and Dental Hypnotherapy Association and the IACT - International Association of Counselors and Therapists

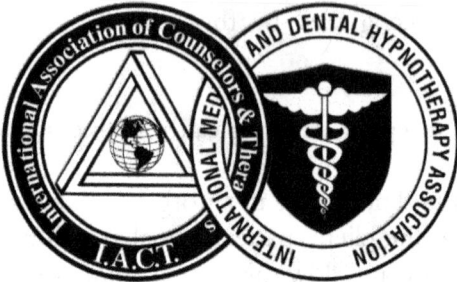

INTRODUCTION by Linda Bennett

"The purpose of life is not to be happy. It is to be useful, to be honorable, to be compassionate, to have it make some difference that you have lived and lived well."
—Ralph Waldo Emerson

Have you ever felt that your life was a complete mess and you were unsure about what to do to fix it? Well, back in the early 90's I was there, and struggling to get a handle on things. A dear friend suggested that I should try hypnosis. Desperate, I decided to give it a try and my life has never been the same since. In the very first session I had, I was so comfortable with the process that it felt as if all of a sudden I belonged. I am not even sure what I believed I belonged to; however, two weeks later I had enrolled in school and was on my way to becoming a hypnotherapist. Now I really belonged. I found that I was a natural and everything about the world of hypnosis made sense to me. It was both logical and creative, and fit me to a T.

Hypnosis has been my life ever since. I love the miracles and magic of what is possible. I find most of us are seeking to change something in our lives and about ourselves, and often give up too soon when making change becomes difficult. Hypnosis helps take the difficulty out of the challenge of instituting much needed change! My life began to improve after that first session. I grew from a troubled woman often considering suicide to an empowered woman loving everything about life.

During my career I had the pleasure of meeting Dan Dziadura, a student that was affiliated with one of our local hospitals. Dan approached me about the possibility of working together on a pain study at the hospital he worked with, and I jumped at the chance. We had a few hurdles to overcome in the process of developing this program; but eventually we got the green light and were able to move full steam ahead. Initially, we were limited to just a few departments in the hospital; as our success became known, we were invited to participate in more and more units, including outpatient surgery and the emergency department.

The participants in our pilot initiative were graduates of the SWIHA - Southwest Institute of Healing Arts hypnotherapy program for which I am the director and one of the instructors. Our participants volunteered their time and were asked to commit to completing 100 hours to the study. Several members of our team were still participating four years after this initiative was implemented, volunteering well over 500 hours individually.

It's been such a joy to witness the impact this program has had on the hospital, their patients, the staff and our graduates. We know we made a difference and we hope this publication might inspire other hospitals to make a difference in a new way.

Through my teaching at SWIHA, I have met thousands of incredible students eager to make a difference in the world. One of those remarkable graduates is Gisele Marasca-Vargas. Gisele is a visionary and an inspiration. She proposed the idea for this publication, and I am so grateful that she is the guide to a project that is destined to make a difference in the world of healing.

Linda Bennett, MS, CCHt, LC

INTRODUCTION by Gisele Marasca-Vargas

I was introduced to hypnotherapy by accident. In 2010, my life had turned upside down. As a consequence of the 2008 economic crisis, among other factors, my business partner and I had to close our graphic design and publishing business. I was forced to declare bankruptcy and lost my home in the process. I had to start over in my 40's, when everything I had believed in or counted on didn't make sense any longer. I was feeling lost, confused, depressed and very angry. After a period of grieving and a short stretch working for the U.S. Census, I came to the realization that I needed to start reinventing myself.

Since 2002, I had been learning about and experimenting with different forms of holistic practices as a side activity. I really enjoyed that work, so I decided to pursue the integrative arts as a career. The research I conducted about federally accredited holistic healthcare programs led me to SWIHA - Southwest Institute of Healing Arts in Tempe, AZ as the best choice for my purposes. In 2011, when I enrolled in the SWIHA AOS degree program in Holistic Health Care (with concentration in Mind Body Transformational Psychology), I had the choice to specialize in nutrition or hypnotherapy. The latter sounded more interesting, so that's the one I picked; and the rest is history.

I had not intended to become a hypno-coach or guided imagery practitioner when I first enrolled in the SWIHA integrative arts program. As most everyone, I had many misconceptions about Guided Imagery/Hypnotherapy and its uses. As I learned more about it, I was quite surprised to discover that my perceptions were simply myths that originated from lack of information and were perpetuated by media (movies, TV shows, stage "hypnotists" and mentalists, etc). Likewise, I was surprised to realize how profoundly effective this simple, natural and non-invasive technique really is.

From that moment on, Hypno-coaching (Hypnotherapy/Guided Imagery combined with Life Coaching) became both my passion and main specialty as a wellness practitioner. Even after many years of practice and several hundreds of clients, it never ceases to amaze me how effective this integrative approach can be for positive transformation on so many levels.

Over the past few years, my clientele has expanded to include traditional healthcare professionals (staff, nurses, department heads, administrators, etc) who have experienced the usual remarkable results from Hypno-coaching sessions for a broad spectrum of issues such as stress and anxiety, depression, anger management, burn-out, fatigue, sleep distress, public speaking, loss and grief, self-esteem, motivation and weight management, among others. One of my clients, a hospital surgeon, was shocked and amazed at how quickly and effectively Guided Imagery/Hypnotherapy released her from a life-limiting phobia; and all it took was a couple of sessions. Another client, a department head at a branch of a major regional hospital group in Orlando, FL, invited me to offer a presentation about hypnotherapy for her department staff, which was well-received. Since then, I have been working with and seeking further opportunities to share information about Guided Imagery/Hypnotherapy at other healthcare facilities. As part of these efforts, I gathered the information and knowledge I had been accumulating, along with additional stats and research, and started working on a book about the effectiveness of hypnotherapy.

Attending the SWIHA hypnotherapy program is also where I was fortunate to meet and learn from my gifted and accomplished instructor and mentor Linda Bennett, Director of the Guided Imagery/Hypnotherapy program at SWIHA. Professor Bennett and Dan Dziadura, PT, DHSc, a hospital director and a SWIHA graduate, partnered to pilot a guided imagery initiative at a major regional hospital in Arizona. Once I learned about the amazing results their initiative has been achieving, it just made sense to combine our information and experiences into a book and spread the word about Guided Imagery/Hypnotherapy; especially taking into consideration how effective this technique has proven to be as a tool to help reduce the stress, fatigue and burn-out in healthcare professionals and patients, recently escalated by the Covid healthcare crisis (please refer to the article interview with Professor Bennett by Paul Gallese, PT, MBA below).

I am deeply honored for having the opportunity to co-author this book with Professor Bennett, and earnestly hope that it will become a useful tool for healthcare professionals and patients everywhere.

Gisele Marasca-Vargas, CCHt, CLC, CWP

Reference:
Helping Caregivers Manage Stress, Burnout and Fatigue. An Interview with Linda Bennett, MS, CCHt, LC, by Paul Gallese, PT, MBA
https://www.vitalacy.com/post/helping-caregivers-manage-stress-burnout-and-fatigue-an-interview-with-linda-bennett-ph-d

CHAPTER 1

WHAT GUIDED IMAGERY/HYPNOTHERAPY IS (AND WHAT IT IS NOT)

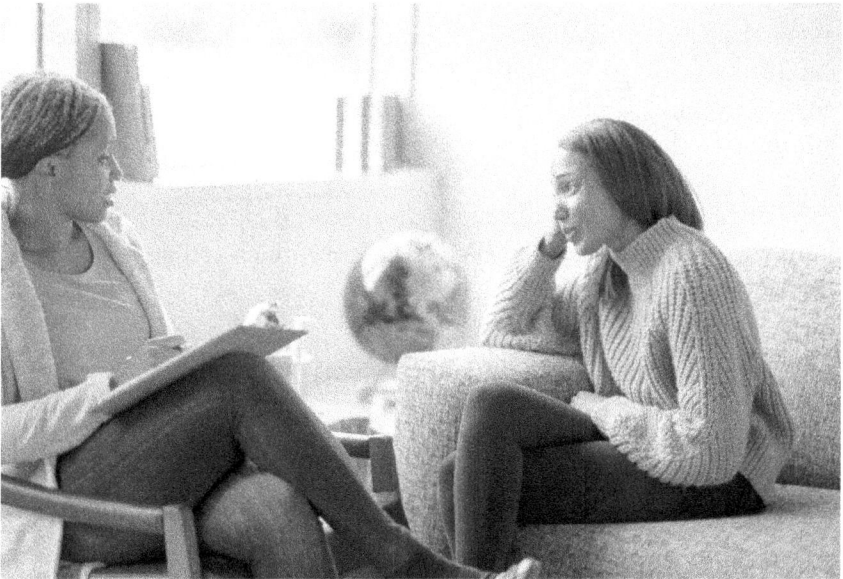

I. What Guided Imagery/Hypnotherapy *Is*:
- Guided Imagery/Hypnotherapy is the use of metaphoric and/or suggestive language to help achieve a natural altered state of mind or trance that's between waking and deep sleep, and is characterized by increased suggestibility, relaxation and heightened imagination. This state is commonly referred to as "zoning out." Through this simple, non-invasive technique, it's possible to make suggestions for positive change on a subconscious level, using the power of the mind. If the mind can visualize positive change and believe it's already happening, it can achieve it.

- Guided Imagery/Hypnotherapy is comparable to guided meditation, creative visualization, Yoga Nidra and other similar non-invasive techniques for promoting relaxation and making it possible to tap into the subconscious mind.

- Guided Imagery/Hypnotherapy usually brings a very pleasant feeling of complete physical and mental relaxation. If you go into a deep trance involving light sleep, once you awake you might not consciously remember everything about the words used during your guided imagery experience. However, it is important to realize that your subconscious mind still remembers everything that is said during that experience. Your subconscious is able to recognize, understand and accept the message, even if your conscious mind doesn't recall all or any of it (similarly to reading out loud without consciously paying attention to the text).

- Positive change and results can occur independently from the individual's awareness or level of relaxation, which can go from lighter to deeper states.

- Most people are capable of reaching a hypnotic state, as long as they are motivated to do so.

II. What Guided Imagery/Hypnotherapy *Is Not*:

1. It's *Not* Mind control
Unlike popular belief, you can't make anyone do anything they don't want to do through Guided Imagery/Hypnotherapy. In reality, any hypnosis is self-hypnosis, even if someone else is facilitating it for you; you are in control and have to agree to the process for it to work.

"While most people fear losing control in hypnosis, it is in fact a means of enhancing mind-body control." —*Dr. David Spiegel, director of the Center on Stress and Health and medical director of the Center for Integrative Medicine at Stanford*

2. It's *Not* Just Going to sleep

As mentioned above, the goal of Guided Imagery/Hypnotherapy is not to make you fall asleep. However, this process also works well during light sleep.

3. It's *Not* Woo Woo or Miracle Cure

Guided Imagery/Hypnotherapy is scientifically based; plenty of studies about its effectiveness for many different uses are available (please refer to **Appendix C:** *Stats & Research About Guided Imagery/Hypnotherapy*).

Guided Imagery/Hypnotherapy is not intended as a therapeutic treatment or replacement for therapeutic treatments.

4. It's *Not* Placebo Effect

Research shows that Guided Imagery/Hypnotherapy works through a change in the brain's perception, as measured by PET/CT - Positron Emission Tomography. In one study, subjects were shown a black and white sample while being guided to believe that they were looking at a color sample. The areas of the brain that recognize color lit up during the test. The opposite was also true (while being shown a color sample, subjects were guided to believe that they were looking at a black and white sample, and the areas of the brain that recognize black and white lit up during the test).

Dr. Spiegel's research has also shown that Guided Imagery/Hypnotherapy can act on multiple brain regions, including some linked to pain perception and regulation. It also quiets parts of the brain involved in sensory processing and emotional response.

Due to rapid advances in the Epigenetics field, several studies are currently available about the genetics of hypnosis, or how Guided Imagery/Hypnotherapy can also change gene expression. In other words, we are what we think. According to the article *On Hypnosis and Genetics* by Afik Faerman, Ph.D., from Stanford University, "Hypnosis can also change how our genetic information comes into play: undergoing hypnosis sessions has been linked to the activation of genetic programs related to a healthy immune response, stem cell growth, reduced inflammation, and decreased stress." For sources and additional information, please refer to **Appendix C:** *Stats & Research About Guided Imagery/Hypnotherapy.*

Of course, as with any therapy, the placebo effect can be achieved by establishing rapport with the facilitator, being given information about the potential positive effects of the technique or procedure, etc; and that can reinforce and enhance the process. Guided Imagery/ Hypnotherapy is, after all, a client-centered technique that focuses on the client's self-empowerment and healing goals.

5. It's *Not* Harmful

Guided Imagery/Hypnotherapy is a safe, natural and non-invasive way to induce relaxation and guide you through positive change. It can be used for pain control/management, but that's advisable to take place only after a doctor has evaluated the person for any physical disorder that might require medical or surgical treatment.

Guided Imagery/Hypnotherapy might not be appropriate for a person who has psychotic symptoms, such as hallucinations and delusions, or for someone who is abusing drugs or alcohol.

III. Guided Imagery/Hypnotherapy FAQs:

1. Does Guided Imagery/Hypnotherapy work better with the weak-minded?

No! In fact, the stronger the will of a person, the more likely they are to achieve success with Guided Imagery/Hypnotherapy. This is because people are most influenced by their own suggestions and, in reality, put themselves into a natural trance state. The facilitator's role is to guide them in this process. As mentioned above, no one can get into this state against their will, or be made to do something they don't want to do.

Guided Imagery/Hypnotherapy actually works as a narrowing or focusing of attention. "Hypnosis is to consciousness what a telephoto lens is to a camera," says Dr. Spiegel.

2. Guided Imagery/Hypnotherapy is very client centered and solution-focused, working with the client's own belief system and intended outcomes.

3. Is it difficult to come out of or wake up from Guided Imagery/ Hypnotherapy?

It is easy to be brought back from a Guided Imagery/Hypnotherapy trance; there has never been a documented case of someone unable to come out of it.

4. Are there any potential risks or dangers with Guided Imagery/ Hypnotherapy?

There is no known risk related to the use of Guided Imagery/ Hypnotherapy for relaxation and other uses.

5. What is Self-Guided Imagery/Hypnotherapy?

Self-Guided Imagery/Hypnotherapy is the self-induced practice of guiding oneself into a natural trance by making use of self-suggestions and affirmations. It can help reinforce the work done during guided sessions. In a way, all Guided Imagery/Hypnotherapy is a form of self-Guided Imagery/Hypnotherapy.

The next chapter addresses Guided Imagery/Hypnotherapy uses in healthcare.

CHAPTER 2

GUIDED IMAGERY/HYPNOTHERAPY
USES IN HEALTHCARE

"In today's society, Guided Imagery/Hypnotherapy as a modality of care is well recognized by the general public and the Health Professions." —*Robert F. Otto, President and CEO of IMDHA and IACT*

The focus of this chapter is on how guided imagery/hypnotherapy is being used today, as well as its potential uses tomorrow.

What can Hypnotherapy be used for?
Hypnotherapy can be of great use for behavioral, physical and psychological conditions such as:

• Allergies

• Anger Management

• Athletic Performance

• Chronic Health Conditions

• Death and Dying

• Depression

• Fears and Phobias

• General Health and Well-being

• GI Conditions

• Insomnia/Sleep Distress

• Learning Disabilities

- Loss and Grief

- Pain Management

- Reaching Life Goals

- Relationship Issues

- Self Esteem and Motivation

- Stress and Anxiety

- Surgery Preparation/Anesthesia

- Weight Management

Meet the IMDHA - International Medical and Dental Hypnotherapy Association:
The IMDHA was founded to familiarize medical professionals and the public with the benefits of Guided Imagery/Hypnotherapy, as well as to provide a resource to connect with well-trained hypnotherapists.
According to the IMDHA, the use of Guided Imagery/Hypnotherapy can "help create a sense of peace and harmony within the individual [patient], so that current medical challenge can be met and dealt with in a positive manner, thus making the procedures towards wellness and peace of mind less traumatic.

The objectives include the following:

1. **Aid the physician** and health care team by preparing the patient for the procedure, thereby enhancing the healing process.

2. **Aid the physician** in bringing the patient to a state of wellness and quality of life.

3. **Reinforce the physician's** "orders" and give suggestions for continued speedy recovery.

4. **Aid the hospital** or health care facility in the performance of their function to: *Meet* the requirements of D.R.G. [Diagnosis-Related

Group] and *Reduce* the amount of drugs the patient would normally require, especially in the control of pain.

5. **Reduce the fear** and anxiety associated with medical procedures as well as catastrophic illness.

6. **Assist the family** in reducing their anxiety - stress relief is needed.

7. **Teach the family members** appropriate **positive suggestions** to reinforce the physician's and hospital staff's efforts on behalf of the patient.

8. **Teach the patient** how to use self-hypnosis after the hospital stay to control pain and aid in his/her healing process."

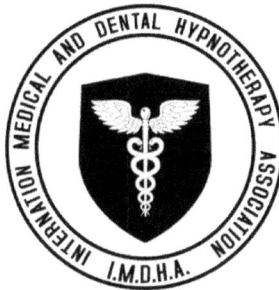

Although there are countless possible uses for Guided Imagery/ Hypnotherapy in the healthcare system, this book will focus primarily on its use for relaxation, stress release, pain management, the reduction of symptoms such as nausea, and a heightened sense of well-being, as demonstrated by the pilot study described in **Chapter 5:** Pilot Study at a Major Regional Hospital in Arizona.

CHAPTER 3

WHY GUIDED IMAGERY/HYPNOTHERAPY?
QUESTIONS AND CONCERNS ADDRESSED

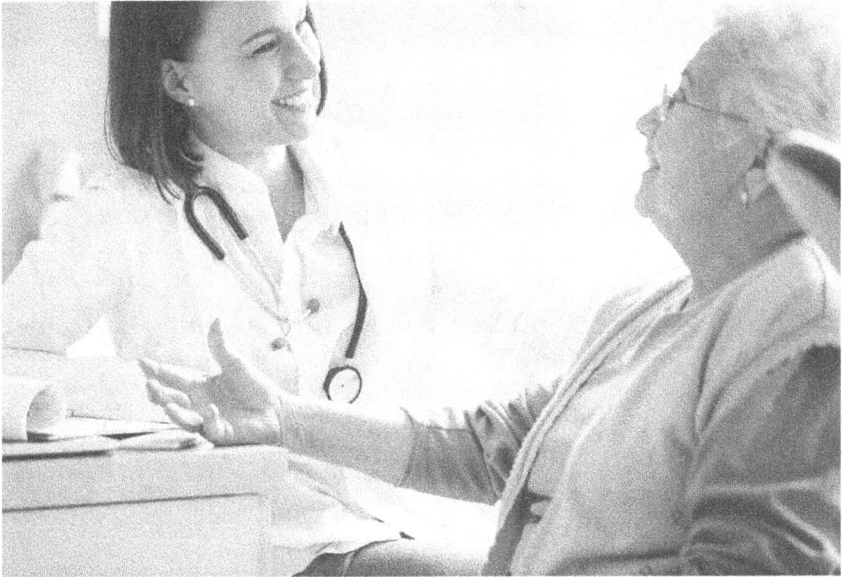

I. Why Guided Imagery/Hypnotherapy?
We'd like to answer this question with another question: Why *not*?

This is an important question, if we consider the following facts:
- The abundance of stats, research and scientific studies that are available about the effectiveness of Guided Imagery/Hypnotherapy for a broad spectrum of physical, emotional and mental issues, especially in comparison with other applied methods (please refer to **Appendix C:** *Stats & Research About Guided Imagery/Hypnotherapy*).

- Guided Imagery/Hypnotherapy can only help; it doesn't cause side effects or harm, as discussed on **Chapter 1:** *What Guided Imagery/Hypnotherapy Is (And What It Is Not).*

- Several hospitals, clinics and other healthcare facilities throughout the U.S. (and the world) have successfully implemented Guided Imagery/Hypnotherapy programs (please refer to **Appendix C:** *Stats & Research About Guided Imagery/Hypnotherapy*).

- Guided Imagery/Hypnotherapy benefits healthcare professionals, staff and patients, with no downside (please refer to **Chapter 5:** *Pilot Study at a Major Regional Hospital in Arizona* and **Appendix A:** *Charts and Graphs from Banner Hospital Surveys*).

- A Guided Imagery/Hypnotherapy program is one of the easiest and most cost-effective programs that can be implemented and maintained at a healthcare facility (please refer to **Chapter 4:** *How to Start a Guided Imagery Program at a Healthcare Facility*).

II. Questions and Concerns About Implementing a Guided Imagery/Hypnotherapy Program:

1. Lack of accurate information about Guided Imagery/Hypnotherapy, which we provide in **Chapter 1:** *What Guided Imagery/Hypnotherapy Is (And What It Is Not).*

2. Lack of knowledge, experience and/or availability of qualified professionals willing to implement and run a Guided Imagery/Hypnotherapy program.

3. The belief that it's expensive to set up and run a Guided Imagery/Hypnotherapy program.

4. The belief that it's too difficult and time-consuming to set up and run a Guided Imagery/Hypnotherapy program.

5. Liability concerns

We address items 2 through 5 in the next three chapters of this book.

CHAPTER 4

PILOT STUDY AT A MAJOR REGIONAL HOSPITAL IN ARIZONA

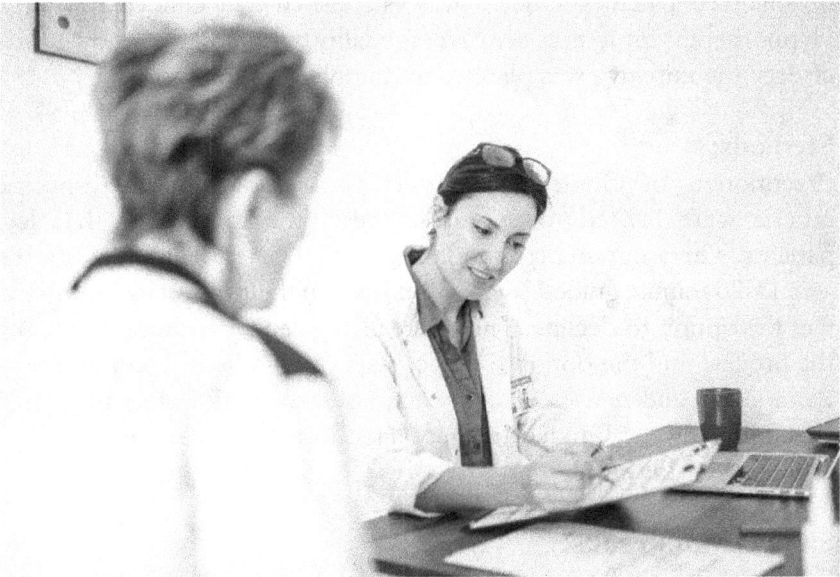

The Effects of Guided Imagery/Hypnotherapy on Pain, Stress and Nausea in Hospitalized Patients

Project Directors:
- **Dan Dziadura,** PT, DHSc, MSPT, Director of Rehabilitation Services, and Wellness Coordinator

- **Linda Bennett,** MS, CCHt, LC, Associate Dean of Education and Director of the Hypnotherapy/Guided Imagery Program at SWIHA - Southwest Institute of Healing Arts.

Background:

Being admitted to a hospital can be a stressful and frightening experience. The goal of the Guided Imagery/Hypnotherapy pilot initiative was to supplement traditional care with an effective non-traditional alternative to help relieve stress and other common symptoms, in addition to facilitating a sense of peace and calm with patients.

A pilot study was formed to assess the use of Guided Imagery/ Hypnotherapy as a tool to manage pain, stress and nausea with hospitalized patients. Once it was established that Guided Imagery/ Hypnotherapy is a non-invasive modality without any known side effects, the initiative was planned and implemented.

Methods:

Practitioners of Guided Imagery/Hypnotherapy who met specific criteria were invited to volunteer their time to work with select patients. The program began in January of 2015. Patients were offered free 15-20 minute guided Imagery sessions in their hospitals rooms and had the option to decline. They were also given a brochure explaining the process and the option to select a script from 5 different choices. Pain, stress and nausea scores were assessed immediately preceding and following the Guided Imagery/Hypnotherapy session, using a 1-10 verbal analog scale.

Summary of Results:

When the project first began, the hospital designated two departments within which volunteers could assist clients with pain management, stress management and nausea levels. Positive results became immediately apparent.

At first there was some skepticism from many of the nursing and medical staff. To address it, meetings and demonstrations were scheduled for the staff to get firsthand experience. A little bit of education can go a long way! Soon the program Project Directors were asked to offer these services to additional departments. Nurses and Doctors alike were asking for Guided Imagery/Hypnotherapy Volunteers to see specific patients.

After only six months, the Project Directors had been able to collect a great deal of encouraging statistics. When the report below was generated (six months after the pilot project was first implemented), the Guided Imagery/Hypnotherapy initiative was running in seven different departments, including the Emergency Department; and the Project Directors had even ventured into the surgery unit, offering Guided Imagery/Hypnotherapy to both pre- and post-surgery patients! Additional branches of the hospital group had also asked the Directors to bring this project to their hospitals, including the MD Anderson Cancer Center.

The success was amazing! During the first six months of this pilot project, 221 patients received a Guided Imagery/Hypnotherapy session, with the following positive results:

• **Pain levels were reduced by 42%**

• **Stress levels were reduced by 52%**

• **Nausea was reduced by 56%**

Please refer to **Appendix A:** Charts and Graphs from the Hospital Pilot Study for more details.

In the next chapter (**Chapter 5:** Starting a Hospital-based Guided Imagery/Hypnotherapy Program) we share tried and tested protocols for implementing a hospital-based Guided Imagery/Hypnotherapy program. In **Chapter 6:** Hospital Stories, we share some of the positive results and personal accounts, as reported by patients, hospital staff and volunteers.

CHAPTER 5

STARTING A HOSPITAL-BASED GUIDED IMAGERY/HYPNOTHERAPY PROGRAM

Please see below the steps taken to implement the pilot program mentioned on the previous chapter. These steps allowed us to develop basic guidelines on how to successfully establish a similar program in your healthcare facility.

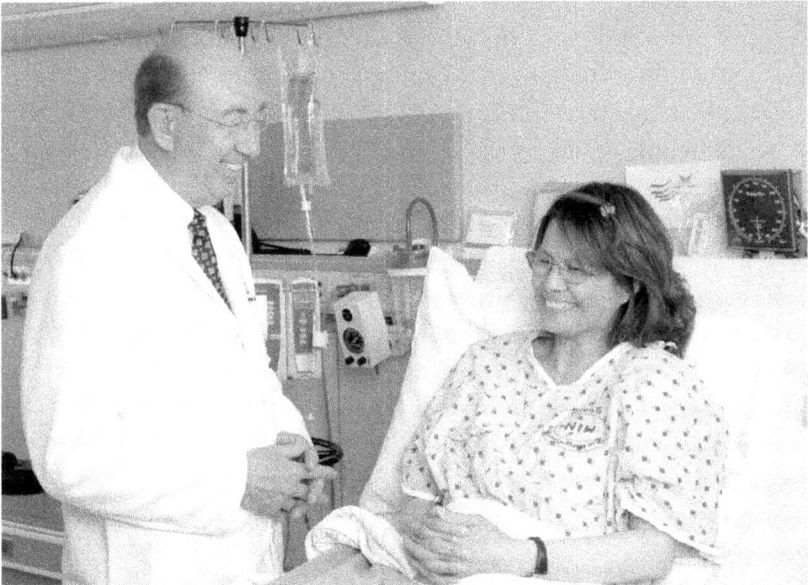

1. Identify all hospital stakeholders and obtain consents and permissions as necessary, including, but not limited to:

    • **Facility Senior Management Team**

    • **Chief Medical Officer**

- **Chief Nursing Officer**

- **Compliance Officer/Risk/Legal team**

- **Volunteer Department Leader (if using volunteers)**

2. Use this booklet as a guide and to share information about implementing a Guided Imagery/Hypnotherapy initiative.

3. If using volunteers: Partner with a federally accredited and reputable educational institution that offers an in-depth hypnotherapy program, such as SWIHA - Southwest Institute of Healing Arts (Tempe, AZ). This program can also be implemented with just nursing and other hospital staff.

4. Determine the minimum acceptable requirements for practitioners.

5. Schedule education sessions for the nursing departments and other staff to generate engagement and gain cooperation among staff members.

6. Create brochures/flyers to educate patients about the Guided Imagery/Hypnotherapy process and potential benefits.

7. Create a Volunteer Application and Agreement for the program (if using volunteers).

8. Create assessment forms, Guided Imagery/Hypnotherapy scripts and other necessary documents.

9. Conduct training for volunteers (or nursing and/or other hospital staff) to ensure that the initiative standards, protocols and other necessary hospital requirements are observed.

10. Establish the procedure for assessment document collection.

CHAPTER 6

HOSPITAL STORIES AND TESTIMONIALS

"So often I see new hypnotherapy and life coaching graduates give up way too easily. I started my career back in the early 1990's. A lot has changed since then and yet it's been an uphill journey. Sometimes the journey has been met with criticism and doubt, and yet I couldn't and wouldn't give up. We may not be the first line of defense for medical care; however, we have started to be noticed and taken seriously. Yes, we can make a difference!' —Linda Bennett, MS, CCHt

From the Hospital Surgery Center Leadership:
"We were so happy to participate in the Guided Imagery trial program. Please pass on our deepest appreciation and respect for the work done by all the volunteers. Their passion for healing was sincerely reflected in the care and attention they showed to our patients. We strongly support the integration of this program into all areas of [major hospital system] and request consideration for the program to be continued at our facility."

From a Patient:
"I had guided imagery this morning and it changed my life. I woke up depressed and an angel came into my room today to show me how to do this at home.
It has opened my eyes and mind. I am going to share this with my family."

Volunteer Experiences
Here are some success stories shared by program volunteers about their Guided Imagery/Hypnotherapy experience with patients and staff:

"I heard a patient moaning, talking very loudly, agitated. She complained about her pain. She couldn't sleep, the hospital staff didn't understand her condition. 'All I want is ice chips or I will throw up and that will hurt so bad.'
The nurse left, I entered introduced myself, explained my role. I listened for about 30 minutes as she vented about all the challenges she was facing. When the patient began to wind down, I offered Guided Imagery. She chose a script. When a nurse came, I told the patient she could answer the nurse, then drift down again. When I finished she was asleep, relaxed physically, breathing comfortably. I let her sleep."

[Guided Imagery/Hypnotherapy Program Volunteer]

"There was a very agitated patient. The patient was struggling to get any sleep and was giving the nurses a challenging time. Patient was willing to give the guided imagery a try. Within moments the patient was in a deep relaxation. All of a sudden an alarm in the room started to sound. I keep on talking, the patient kept on relaxing and finally a nurse came in an addressed the cause of the alarm. After I completed the imagery exercise I mentioned the alarm and the patient looked at me with surprise and said "what alarm?" This was coming from someone who had been unable to get some sleep!"

[Guided Imagery/Hypnotherapy Program Volunteer]

From the few pre-surgery patients I have seen, I have a very strong sense that doing imagery before surgery is one of areas we really can contribute to. I've also surmised that patients in pain are willing to try anything that might help. They are very quick to agree to imagery within minutes) and are surprised to see their pain does decrease or disappear in twenty minutes. During the healing story she seemed to relax, her lips parted periodically and her breathing seemed slower and rhythmic. Afterwards, she appeared very relaxed and comfortable and mentioned what a good experience she had. The doctor arrived within minutes of ending the story and said that her heart rate had gone from about 146 to 128! The nurse outside the room could see the numbers descending on the machine as I was doing the imagery. Prior to the story, the patient's pain and stress levels were in the 3s and 4s and they reduced 1-2 points."

[Guided Imagery/Hypnotherapy Program Volunteer]

"As I explained the Guided Imagery to Jennifer and mentioned one of the stories included "floating on a cloud," she lit up and expressed her love of Angles. At that moment, I knew who I had brought my *Angel Music* CD for!

At the end of the session, Jennifer was shedding some tears and also thanking me for the 'beautiful experience.' She told me her daughter in law, who had passed away a few years ago, was there with her at the healing place [from the Guided Imagery script]. I stayed a while longer while she expressed what was on her mind…and in her heart.

It was an angelic experience for Jennifer…and a special experience for me. Of course…her stress and pain numbers went down!"

[Guided Imagery/Hypnotherapy Program Volunteer]

"I had a patient who had his leg amputated and was in pain and not doing well. He was referred to me by his nurse. We finished the script and he cried with an emotional release. He said the script was beautiful and he saw himself walking down the path alongside the stream.

He asked me to come back in 10 minutes. When I came back he looked refreshed and smiling, he had shaved and cleaned up. We talked about his 17 yrs as an airline attendant. He was smiling as he spoke.

2.5 hours spent with him talking. He said he forgot all about that his leg was missing during that time.

To sum it up, the program allows me to use my gifts to listen and show compassion for a brief moment in a patient's life during difficult times. I am grateful."

[Guided Imagery/Hypnotherapy Program Volunteer]

"My Incredible Experience

I approached the door and gently knocked. I slowly pushed open the door and the beautiful bald woman laying in the hospital bed smiled at me. She looked exhausted but she managed to smile at me.

I explained guided imagery to the woman and how it may benefit her, and help to feel more relaxed and experience less pain. The woman agreed to a session. I did a session using the Waterfall Script because the woman said she wanted to relax and get rid of some of the pain, nausea and anxiety. We did the intake form. I recorded her numbers. We did the session.

25

As the session came to a close and the woman opened her eyes, she picked up her hands and, staring at her hands, started saying 'My hands, my hands.' I was not sure what she meant and I gently asked her if everything was okay. But the woman kept repeating 'My hands, My hands.' I was about to turn around and go get a nurse when the woman looked me in the eyes and said, 'Look at this,' as she pulled the bed sheet back from her feet. She was wiggling her toes. 'I suffer from Neuropathy of the hands and feet from all of the chemo. I have not been able to wiggle or feel my toes or fingers without pain for weeks. I am wiggling my fingers and toes without pain and I can feel them!' This incredible woman proceeded to tell me she had a double mastectomy earlier that day.

I explained to the woman that this is a place and this is a feeling she can come back to at any time she chooses just by thinking about it and imagining it. It is her place to go to, to guide her along her healing journey. When I did the outtake, every number went down to 0.

Before I left, the woman expressed that she wished everyone could experience this and that she hoped that 'Everyone on the fifth floor could experience this miracle.' "

[Guided Imagery/Hypnotherapy Program Volunteer]

What This Project Means to the Volunteers: "We Can Make a Difference!"

"What the project means to me: This is an important opportunity to demonstrate objectively the benefits Guided Imagery/Hypnosis can bring to hospital patients and the staff, improving the well-being of both groups."

[Guided Imagery/Hypnotherapy Program Volunteer]

"As far as my experience at [major hospital branch], as the pilot unfolds, I continue to have a huge appreciation for the process and find myself experiencing awe and wonderment in what can be accomplished in a mere twenty minutes of imagery. 'Will someone please pinch me?' periodically comes to mind. Sometimes I see the wonderment or confusion on the patient's faces right after. They're not exactly sure what happened, though they sure like the results!"

[Guided Imagery/Hypnotherapy Program Volunteer]

"I had an amazing session a couple of weeks ago doing Guided Imagery for the project at [major hospital branch]. This was such a powerful experience for me. It actually kind of rattled me, in a good way. I got to see first hand the incredible power of the mind. It was so beautiful. I will never forget the woman's name nor will I forget her face. It helped me to even more clearly define my path and how I want to use Hypnotherapy moving forward."

[Guided Imagery/Hypnotherapy Program Volunteer]

"I clearly see how effective Guided Imagery can be when offered in conjunction with the regular treatments and medications.

For people to be able to experience relief from the pain and other symptoms due to treatments for cancer and other ailments, even if it is temporary, it is amazing. Teaching people that they can experience this and use these techniques, and they can summon this whenever they want is so amazing.

Thank you for this amazing opportunity to share guided imagery with those who need it the most."

"To sum it up, the program allows me to use my gifts to listen and show compassion for a brief moment in a patient's life during difficult times. I am grateful."

[Guided Imagery/Hypnotherapy Program Volunteer]

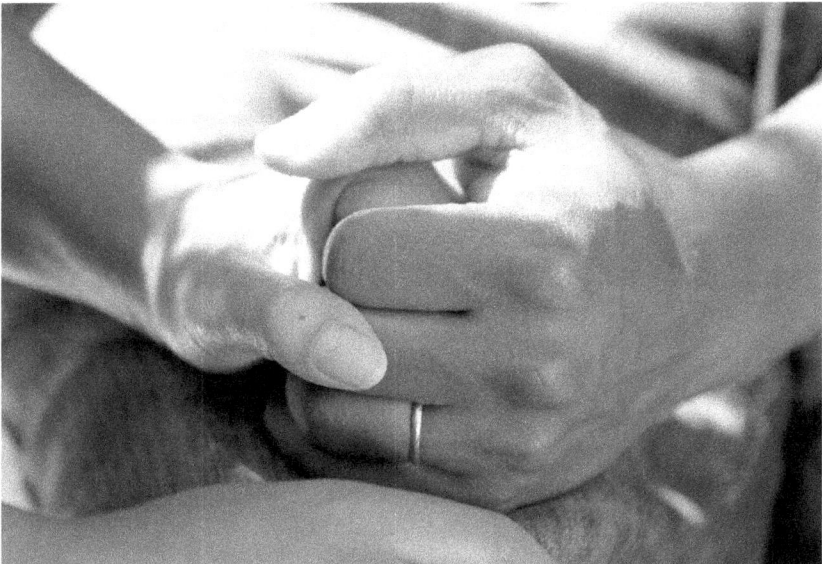

APPENDIX A

CHARTS AND GRAPHS

I. Patient Studies on Stress, Pain and Nausea Reduction:

Mean Scores - All Units
N = 221
(156 female, 65 male)

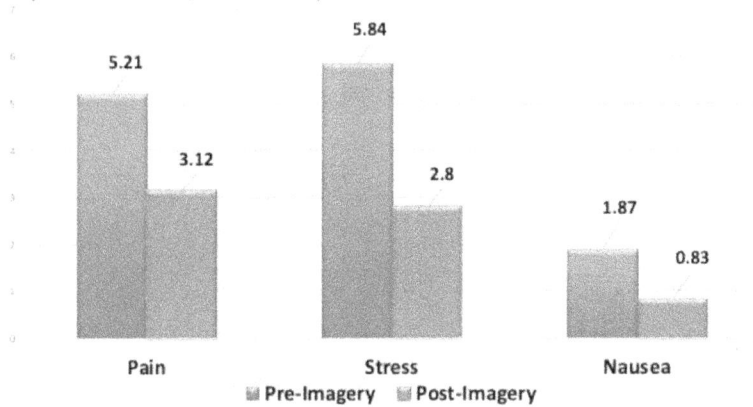

	Pain	Stress	Nausea
Pre-Imagery	5.21	5.84	1.87
Post-Imagery	3.12	2.8	0.83

Pre-Imagery Post-Imagery

Mean Pain Scores by Unit

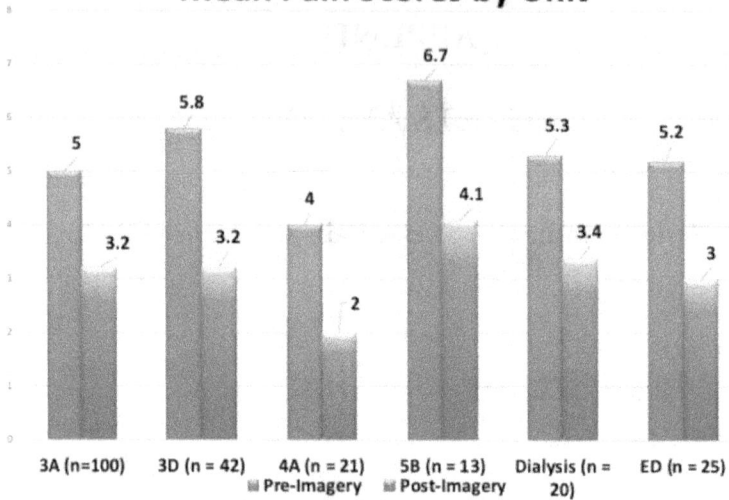

Bar chart showing Pre-Imagery and Post-Imagery mean pain scores by unit:

- 3A (n=100): Pre-Imagery 5, Post-Imagery 3.2
- 3D (n = 42): Pre-Imagery 5.8, Post-Imagery 3.2
- 4A (n = 21): Pre-Imagery 4, Post-Imagery 2
- 5B (n = 13): Pre-Imagery 6.7, Post-Imagery 4.1
- Dialysis (n = 20): Pre-Imagery 5.3, Post-Imagery 3.4
- ED (n = 25): Pre-Imagery 5.2, Post-Imagery 3

Legend: Pre-Imagery, Post-Imagery

Mean Stress Scores by Unit

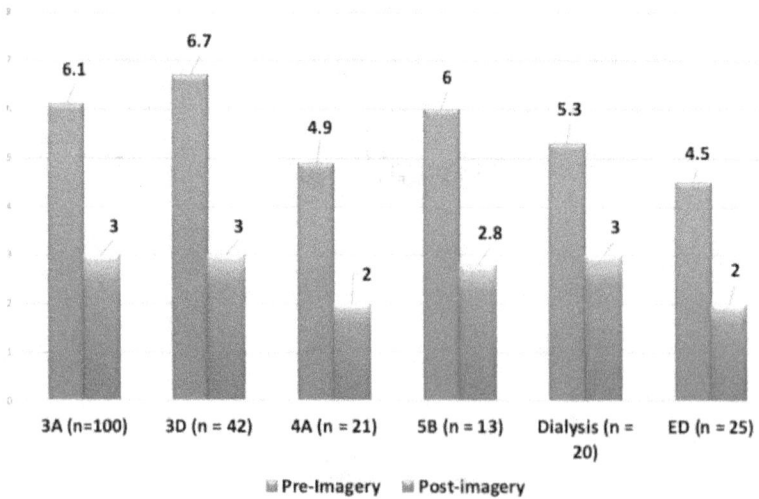

Bar chart showing Pre-Imagery and Post-imagery mean stress scores by unit:

- 3A (n=100): Pre-Imagery 6.1, Post-imagery 3
- 3D (n = 42): Pre-Imagery 6.7, Post-imagery 3
- 4A (n = 21): Pre-Imagery 4.9, Post-imagery 2
- 5B (n = 13): Pre-Imagery 6, Post-imagery 2.8
- Dialysis (n = 20): Pre-Imagery 5.3, Post-imagery 3
- ED (n = 25): Pre-Imagery 4.5, Post-imagery 2

Legend: Pre-Imagery, Post-imagery

30

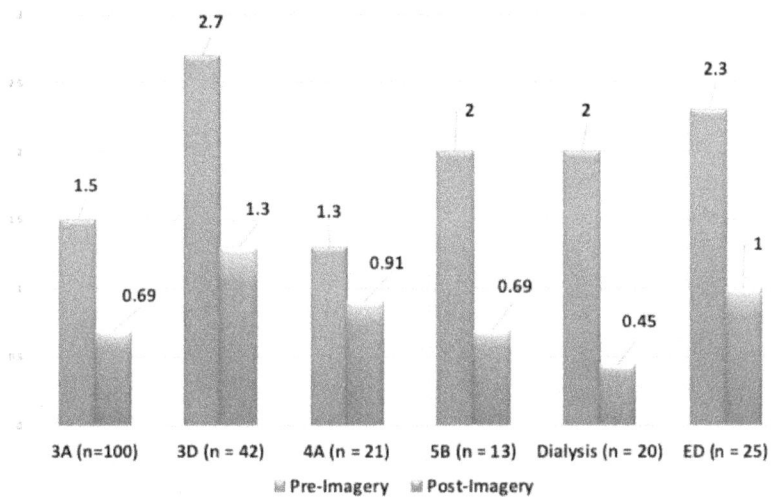

Mean Nausea Scores by Unit

3A (n=100): Pre-Imagery 1.5, Post-Imagery 0.69
3D (n = 42): Pre-Imagery 2.7, Post-Imagery 1.3
4A (n = 21): Pre-Imagery 1.3, Post-Imagery 0.91
5B (n = 13): Pre-Imagery 2, Post-Imagery 0.69
Dialysis (n = 20): Pre-Imagery 2, Post-Imagery 0.45
ED (n = 25): Pre-Imagery 2.3, Post-Imagery 1

Pre-Imagery   Post-Imagery

II. Patients' Viewpoints About the Guided Imagery/Hypnotherapy Program:

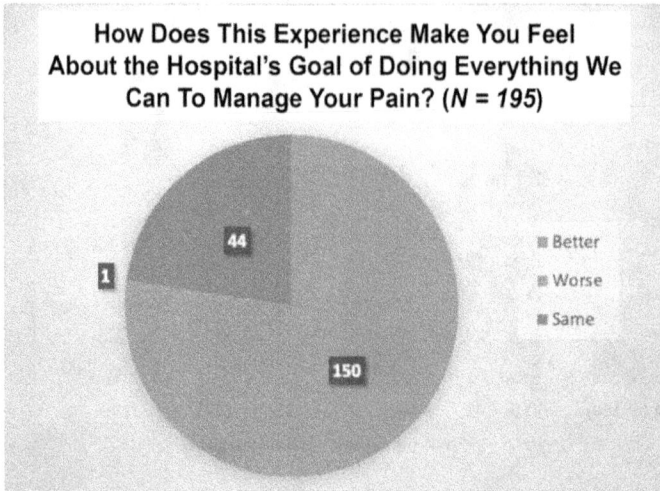

How Does This Experience Make You Feel About the Hospital's Goal of Doing Everything We Can To Manage Your Pain? (N = 195)

- Better
- Worse
- Same

44
1
150

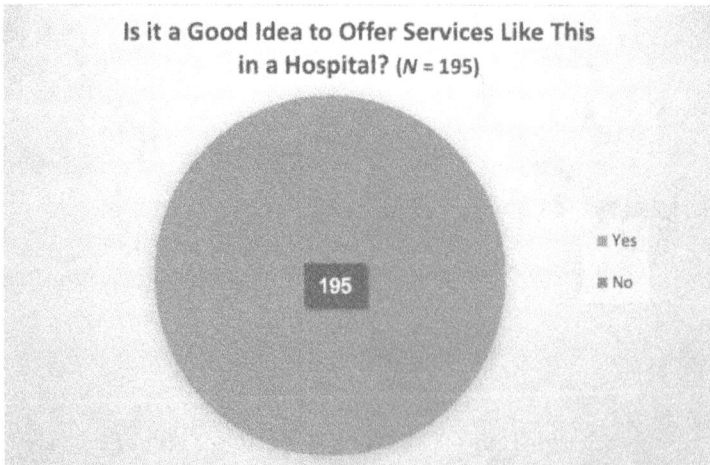

Is it a Good Idea to Offer Services Like This in a Hospital? (N = 195)

- Yes
- No

195

APPENDIX B

STATS AND RESEARCH ABOUT
GUIDED IMAGERY/HYPNOTHERAPY

"While most people fear losing control in hypnosis, it is in fact a means of enhancing mind-body control."
"Hypnosis is to consciousness what a telephoto lens is to a camera."
—*Dr. David Spiegel, Director of the Center on Stress and Health and*
Medical Director of the Center for Integrative Medicine at Stanford

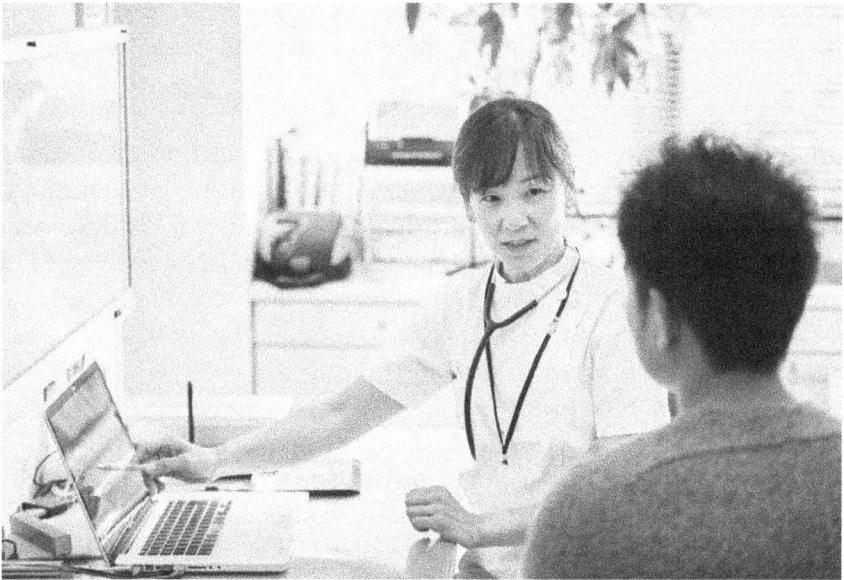

Sampling of Available Studies About Guided Imagery/Hypnotherapy for Anxiety/Stress, Pain, Nausea and Other Conditions:
- Many studies have found Guided Imagery/Hypnotherapy and Self-Hypnosis to be a fast, cost-effective, non-addictive and safe alternative

to medication for the treatment of **anxiety- and stress-related conditions**. For instance, according to Donald Robertson's article (Hypnosis Research & Evidence, 2004), "in a research study involving over 100 patients suffering from stress-related conditions it was found that 75% felt their symptoms were improving after 12 weeks of self-hypnosis practice, within one year 72% of the group reported complete remission of their symptoms as a result of the self-hypnosis (Maher-Loughnan, G.P. 1980, *Hypnosis: Clinical application of hypnosis in medicine*, British Journal of Hospital Medicine, 23: 447-55)."

- "Generally speaking, literature review supports the value of Hypnosis in **analgesia and stress reduction** in a number of disorders, whether following the dissociative formulation (Miller, 1986) or a social psychology approach (Noland, 1987)." (Mentioned on the *High Blood Pressure or Hypertension*; under **References**.)

- "In one study, Guy H. Montgomery, PHD and colleagues tested the effectiveness of a 15-minute pre-surgery hypnosis session versus an empathic listening session in a clinical trial with 200 breast cancer patients.

In a 2007 article in the Journal of the National Cancer Institute (Vol. 99, No. 17), the team reported that patients who received hypnosis reported less **post-surgical pain, nausea, fatigue and discomfort**. The study also found that the hospital saved $772 per patient in the hypnosis group, mainly due to reduced surgical time. Patients who were hypnotized required less of the analgesic lidocaine and the sedative propofol during surgery" (*Hypnosis Today* article; under **References**).

- "How it works: Hypnosis can help you cope with **pain** and gain more self-control over your pain. Additionally, studies indicate that hypnosis can do this effectively for long periods of time" (*6 Surprising Health Benefits Of Hypnosis* Article; under **References**).

- "Kuttner (1988) found that a Hypnotic approach emphasizing storytelling and imagery was significantly more effective than behavioral techniques or standard medical practice in alleviating **distress** during bone marrow aspirations in young children with leukemia." (Mentioned on the *High Blood Pressure or Hypertension*; under **References.**)

- "Hypertensive subjects were found to have characteristic patterns of increased cerebral blood flow that were most marked in the left hemisphere. During Hypnosis, they could reduce **cerebral blood flow** more dramatically than could normotensive controls. The changes noted in this research by Galeazzi (1982) were associated with decreases in **vascular resistance and diastolic blood pressure** in the rest of the body." (Mentioned on the *High Blood Pressure or Hypertension*; under **References**.)

- "Friedman and Taub (1977, 1978) reported the results of a trial comparing Hypnosis with biofeedback or a combination of both in essential **hypertension**. At the end of four weeks of treatment, all groups showed a significant reduction in blood pressure. But at six-month follow-up only the patients receiving Hypnosis had maintained the reduction." (Mentioned on the *High Blood Pressure or Hypertension*; under **References**.)

- Stanford Health Care, the Mayo Clinic and many other reputable hospitals and clinics across the U.S. acknowledge Guided Imagery/ Hypnotherapy as a viable form of treatment for **numerous conditions**. Multiple professional associations have also been promoting Guided Imagery/Hypnotherapy for decades and funding research that continues to prove the effectiveness and countless benefits of Guided Imagery/Hypnotherapy (please see the additional stats and research articles under **References**).

- According to the article *On Hypnosis and Genetics* by Afik Faerman, Ph.D., from Stanford University (under **References**), "Hypnosis can also change how our genetic information comes into play: undergoing hypnosis sessions has been linked to the activation of genetic programs related to a healthy immune response, stem cell growth, reduced inflammation, and decreased stress."

References:

Hypnotherapy is More Mainstream Than You Think
https://web.wellness-institute.org/blog/hypnotherapy-is-more-mainstream-than-you-think

Miscellaneous Medical Applications of Hypnosis
http://www.triroc.com/sunnen/topics/medap.htm

Pilot Study on Epigenetic Response to A Mind-Body Treatment
https://www.ncbi.nlm.nih.gov/pmc/articles/PMC6067070/

On Hypnosis and Genetics
https://www.reveri.com/genes

Hypnosis in the treatment of anxiety- and stress-related disorders
http://www.ncbi.nlm.nih.gov/pubmed/20136382

Hypnosis and the Alleviation of Clinical Pain: A Comprehensive Meta-Analysis
https://www.tandfonline.com/doi/abs/10.1080/00207144.2021.1920330?journalCode=nhyp20

HYPNOSIS FOR ACUTE PROCEDURAL PAIN: A Critical Review
https://www.ncbi.nlm.nih.gov/pmc/articles/PMC5120961/

Hypnotic Approaches for Chronic Pain Management
https://www.ncbi.nlm.nih.gov/pmc/articles/PMC4465776/

Hypnosis and Therapy for a Case of Vomiting, Nausea, and Pain
https://www.tandfonline.com/doi/abs/10.1080/00029157.2015.1040298

Effects of Hypnosis on GI Problems
https://www.med.unc.edu/ibs/wp-content/uploads/sites/450/2017/10/IBS-and-Hypnosis.pdf

High Blood Pressure or Hypertension
https://www.changingstates.co.uk/issues/hypertension.html

Mental Health and Hypnosis
http://www.webmd.com/anxiety-panic/guide/mental-health-hypnotherapy

Stanford Health Care on Medical Hypnosis
https://stanfordhealthcare.org/medical-treatments/h/hypnosis.html

Study Identifies Brain Areas Altered During Hypnotic Trances
https://med.stanford.edu/news/all-news/2016/07/study-identifies-brain-areas-altered-during-hypnotic-trances.html

Hypnosis in Contemporary Medicine
https://www.mayoclinicproceedings.org/article/S0025-6196%2811%2963203-5/fulltext

Mayo Clinic on Hypnosis
https://www.mayoclinic.org/tests-procedures/hypnosis/about/pac-20394405

Research in Hypnotherapy
https://mindbasedhealing.org/research-hypnotherapy/

Hypnosis Research & Evidence, by Donald Robertson (2004)
http://www.ukhypnosis.com/hypnosis-research-evidence/

6 Surprising Health Benefits of Hypnosis
https://www.pennmedicine.org/updates/blogs/health-and-wellness/2019/january/hypnosis

Hypnosis today
https://www.apa.org/monitor/2011/01/hypnosis

DISCLAIMER: *No contraindications of the use of Guided Imagery/ Hypnotherapy for the relief of stress, pain, nausea and other conditions have been found. However, hypnotherapy should not replace care and treatment provided by a medical professional.*

APPENDIX C

GUIDED IMAGERY/HYPNOTHERAPY DEMO SCRIPT

SCRIPT # 4: The Gifts of Healing

To begin with, allow yourself to get comfortable ….. take in a nice big deep breath, and as you release it imagine the tension beginning to leave your body…..

Use the highlighted words if you are working with dialysis patients:
As we continue …. Should you become aware of any sounds… like a motor running, a pump, whistling sounds, alarms… any of those sounds will help you to relax even more, knowing that everything is working exactly as it should… to help you heal and feel stronger… letting the nursing staff take care of you in their expert way…. And as you continue to relax you know how important it is to keep your arm still….. which you will find is easy and comfortable for you to do….

Now with your eyes closed…… focus your attention at the bottoms of your feet….. imagine that there are cords going from the soles of your feet down into the earth…. Grounding you… connecting you…. Imagine that there is now a stream of liquid relaxation flowing up through the center of those cords….. into the soles of your feet…… imagine that this liquid relaxation is now spreading throughout the bottoms of your feet…. Relaxing you…. Feeling very calm and peaceful …. Any outside noises that you may become aware of will simply help you relax more and more……...that liquid relaxation is now spreading…………spreading to the tops of your feet….. your ankles…… relaxing you even more …. You sink deeper and deeper down…..continuing to focus on this pleasant feeling, the liquid relaxation now spreads through your shins….. your calves…… your knees…… your thighs….. your legs are feeling very relaxed now…..

sinking deeper and deeper down….. that liquid relaxation is now flowing through your hips…. Your pelvis …… your stomach….. feeling very relaxed…… it feels so good to just let go and allow this liquid relaxation to spread throughout your body…. Through every nerve… cell….organ and muscle……that liquid relaxation is now flowing into your chest …. Filling your heart and lungs…. Allowing you to breath deeper and feel even more relaxed….. now that liquid relaxation is spreading to your shoulders….. softening all the muscles there in your shoulders…. It might even feel like a great weight has just been lifted from your shoulders…… relaxing even more…. Sinking deeper down….. the liquid relaxation now spreads from your shoulders down through your back… softening each and every muscle in your back……now that liquid relaxation spreads from your shoulders down through each arm….down through your elbows…. Your forearms…… your wrists…. Your hands….. all the way down through your fingertips….. so calm…. so peaceful….. the liquid relaxation is now spreading through your neck and throat….. through your chin and jaw…. Through your cheeks….. behind your eyes….. through your forehead and the top of your head…. Every part of your face is completely relaxed now…in fact, your entire body…. from the tips of your toes, to the top of your head, is filled with this wonderful liquid relaxation….

As you continue to relax, I'd like you to focus on the health challenges you have been experiencing….. There have been moments where you may have felt overwhelmed and frustrated with the stress of the illness… often struggling with finding ways to heal…. And there comes a point where healing can be enhanced with the help of others…. You have now found yourself in a place to receive assistance with your challenges….

Many of us have been taught that it is better to give than to receive…. And because of that belief we often are reluctant to receive what is being offered…instead, we try to do everything ourselves and resist the helping hand being extended to us…… Did you know that there is also a tremendous opportunity to give when we receive?... There are many people… doctors… nurses and hospital staff that are eager to give their knowledge and expertise to you… they are eager to help you feel better and to heal…. They truly want to assist you in feeling better and thriving……..

Imagine that you have been invited to a very special party…. It's a healing party….as you enter this special place where the party is being held, you are warmed by the welcoming individuals who are offering you their gifts…. Each member of the group has something special and unique to offer you… each one is reaching out to you, offering their gifts to help you…… they have dedicated much of their lives to developing their gifts and are eager to share their special healing gifts with you…. At first you might seem overwhelmed…. and then slowly you begin to accept each gift offered… as you accept their gifts, you acknowledge them with appreciation and gratitude…………..as you receive each gift, you allow yourself to receive the benefit that each gift offers…

Imagine what it would look like to receive the gift of pain relief… how would it feel to be pain-free?… Imagine receiving the gift of abundant energy… how would it feel to be strong and clear-minded?… Imagine receiving the gift of feeling great every day… how would it feel to be free of nausea?… free of fatigue and muscle cramps?….

As you open yourself to healing, you begin to allow yourself to receive the healing that is coming from these gifts…. Kind words and encouragement are accompanying each of these gifts… and as you allow yourself to accept the healing being offered, you begin to notice a change coming over you…. You are receiving the gift of healing and comfort……..You also recognize you are giving these wonderful people here the opportunity to give their gifts to you…. You are both giving and receiving…… together the giving and receiving becomes a circle of wholeness and healing……… And it's wonderful to share in this exchange…

Again you thank all these special people for what they are offering you and let them know that you will continue to allow the benefits of their gifts to assist you for the days, weeks, months and years to come…. There is a wonderful quote that reminds us of this experience: "I would maintain that thanks are the highest form of thought; and that gratitude is happiness doubled by wonder"…

The struggle ends when the gratitude begins.... now is the time to be in gratitude for the comfort and healing that you are now receiving.....
As you continue to enjoy this pleasant feeling ... allowing you mind... your body... your spirit to be in complete harmony... perfectly relaxed and calm...from this moment forward.... you are experiencing the many gifts of healing... and you will be able to recall this feeling anytime you choose.... Simply think or say the words thank you and you will be able to return to this calm, relaxed and grateful place.....
Now, with a deep breath, I want you to allow all feeling to return to your body.... Feeling yourself becoming more aware.... and with each breath you are feeling more comfortable.... Alert and refreshed.... Eyes wide open.... fully present now...

Created by Linda Bennett, MS, CCHt, LC

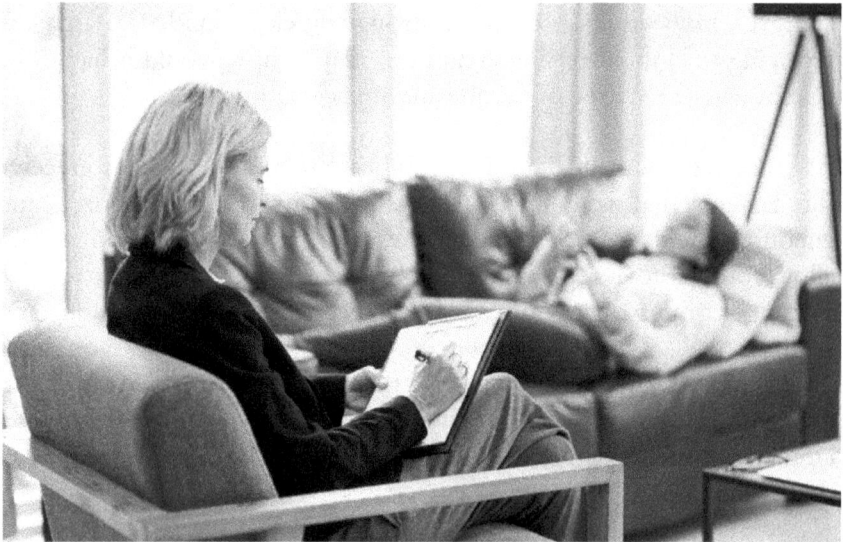

AUTHOR'S BIO

Linda Bennett

Linda Bennett, MS, CCHt, LC is a Certified Clinical Hypnotherapist, Board Certified Hypnotherapy Instructor and Certifying Examiner, as well as a Certified Life Coach. She is the Senior Curriculum Specialist and Hypnotherapy and Guided Imagery Program Director at SWIHA - Southwest Institute of Healing Arts.

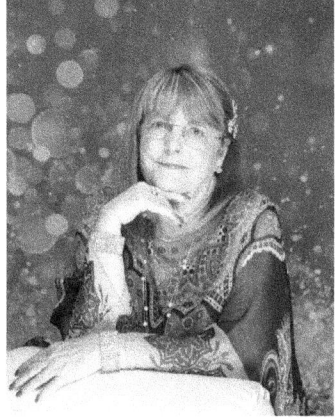

Linda is also the co-founder of Heart Symbol Publishing, which is dedicated to the publication of books and media that inspire, transform and heal the mind, body and spirit (heartsymbolpublishing.com).

Linda is the esteemed 2014 IMDHA - International Medical & Dental Hypnosis Association *Educator of the Year*. She also received the NATH - National Association of Transpersonal Hypnotherapists 2011 *Outstanding Clinical Contribution* Award and the 2022 *Lifetime Achievement* Award, and was recognized for "Outstanding Creativity in the Classroom" for 2005-2006 by the Arizona Private Schools Association. In addition, Linda and her associate Sherry Gilbert were awarded the 2017 and 2022 IMDHA Chapter of the Year for Exceptional Growth & Outreach for Practitioners in the Community.

AUTHOR'S BIO

Gisele Marasca-Vargas

Gisele Marasca-Vargas, CCHt, CLC, CWP obtained her AOS degree in Holistic Healthcare at SWIHA. She is certified as a Master Hypnotherapist through the ABH - American Board of Hypnotherapy and as a Certified Hypno-therapist through the IMDHA - International Medical & Dental Hypnosis Association. Gisele's vision is to help promote well-being from an integrative perspective, and to serve as a channel for healing, awareness, self-empowerment and education. She is the founder of The Healers Home (thehealershome.com; formerly The Ragi Center for Self-Awareness), through which she practices Clinical Hypnotherapy, Life Coaching and other holistic modalities, and offers corporate workshop series and educational presentations about hypno-therapy for the local healthcare community. She also teaches online classes at SWIHA - Southwest Institute of Healing Arts.

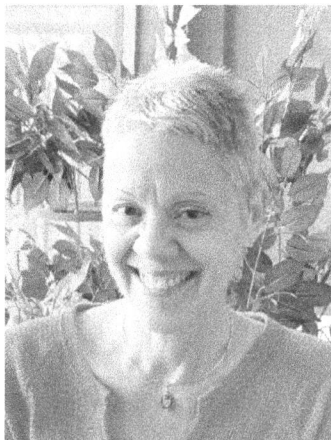

Gisele has a BA in English and Portuguese Languages and an AS in Commercial Art. She was the co-owner of Creative Angle Media, a graphic design and publishing company with several clients in the metro Orlando area, and co-publisher of the award-winning *Ahora/Now* Orlando magazine (a semi-annual bilingual magazine that showcased and played an influencer's role for the Orlando's Hispanic community for seven years). Gisele also writes and blogs (giscreations.com), and is in the process of creating a cat rescue nonprofit organization (giscritters.com). Gisele is originally from São Paulo, Brazil and currently lives with her husband Raul and a number of companion and rescue cats in Orlando, FL.

To order *Guided Imagery/Hypnotherapy for Healthcare: We Can Make a Difference* book copies, additional guided imagery/hypnotherapy scripts or training materials; or to book training workshops for staff and volunteers:

L_GPublishing@yahoo.com or heartcoach@msn.com

NOTES

NOTES

NOTES

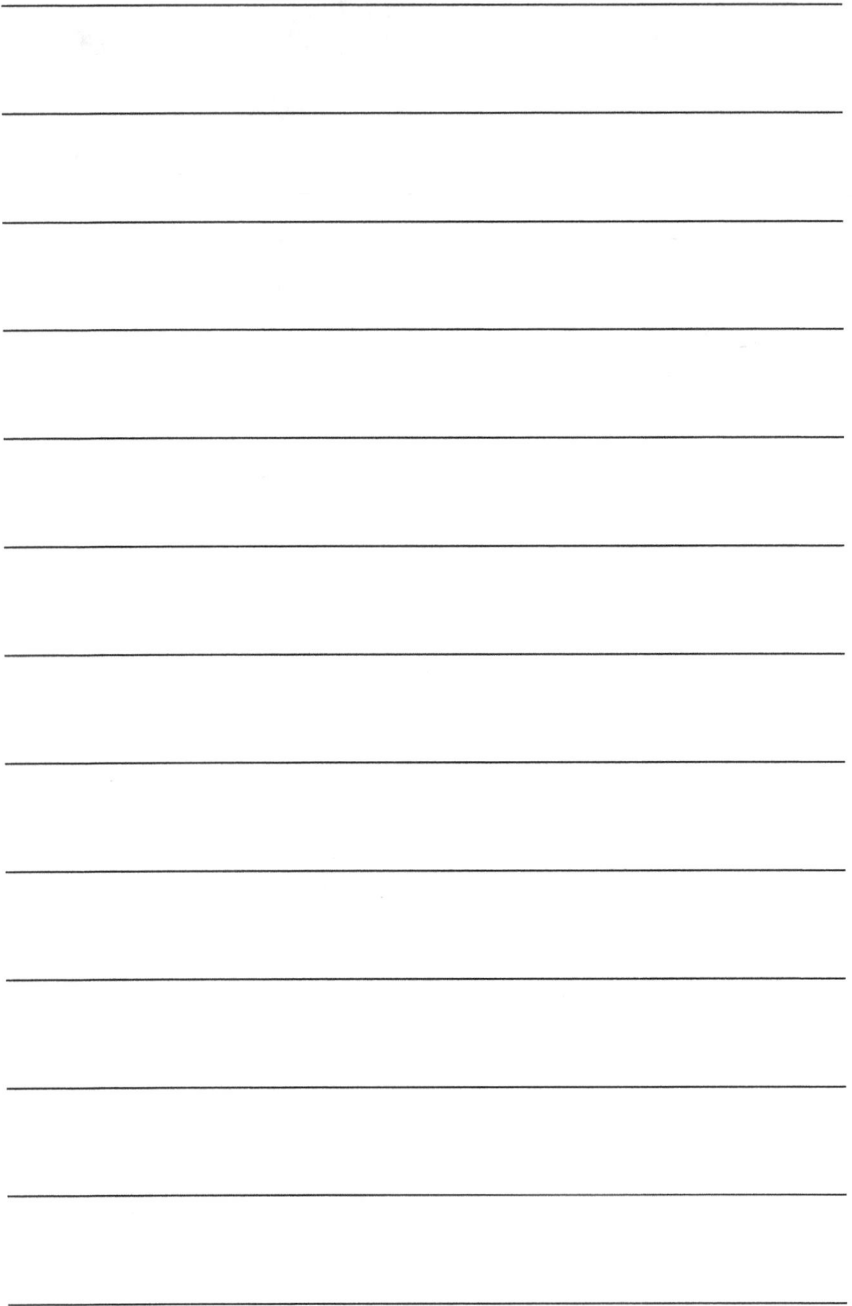

www.ingramcontent.com/pod-product-compliance
Lightning Source LLC
Chambersburg PA
CBHW072211270326
41930CB00011B/2612